UNDERSTANDING SIBO

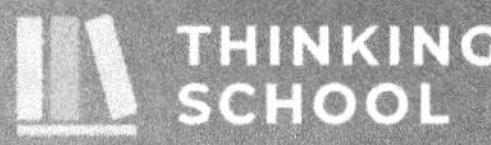

SUSAN MCDOWELL

THINKING SCHOOL

UNDERSTANDING SIBO

The Enigma of Small Intestinal Bacterial Overgrowth

- Susan McDowell -

Understanding SIBO / Susan McDowell – 1st Edition

ISBN 9798321324042

INDEX

INTRODUCTION

Before starting the introduction itself, I want to comment that all the information around SIBO is a living field with more studies concerning this syndrome.

I want this book to be a snapshot of that life, and so I have recently updated the content to add a specific chapter on the SIBO diet.

Let us get started.

SIBO (small intestinal bacterial overgrowth) is a condition that has gained notoriety recently, although it is not new. SIBO is not usually severe. It is characterized by an excess of bacteria in the small intestine, bacteria that normally reside in the large intestine, creating an imbalance in the body.

Diet and lifestyle habits are crucial for preventing SIBO, although there are also uncontrollable factors such as gastrointestinal alterations or anatomical abnormalities. The most common symptoms include abdominal bloating, constipation, flatulence, heartburn, and slow digestion. In severe cases, there may be diarrhea and nutrient absorption problems.

Diagnosis is commonly made through a bacterial overgrowth test, which measures the concentrations of hydrogen and methane in the breath after ingesting a glucose-rich substance.

Treatment varies depending on the patient, but a diet low in fermentable foods, especially sugars and carbohydrates, is generally recommended.

Antibiotics are also used to control the bacterial flora, and probiotics are used to maintain an optimal internal balance.

Emphasis is placed on the importance of maintaining an internal balance of bacteria, known as the microbiota, which is essential for nutrient absorption and the overall functioning of the body. Although SIBO is not usually severe, it is advisable to consult a specialist if symptoms persist.

That is the main reason that In this fascinating book, we will explore the amazing world of our digestive system and learn how to keep it in balance for optimal health and wellness. Our digestive system is much more than just a mechanism for processing food; it is a complex and dynamic ecosystem made up of billions of bacteria, known as the gut microbiota, which plays a crucial role in our overall health.

One of the central topics of this book is SIBO, Small Intestinal Bacterial Overgrowth, a disorder that affects a considerable number of people and can trigger a variety of uncomfortable symptoms and digestive problems. We will explore in depth what SIBO is, its causes, risk factors and diagnostic methods, giving you a solid understanding of this condition.

But we will not only dwell on SIBO, as our approach is holistic and all-encompassing. We will uncover the close relationship between SIBO and other health conditions, such as autoimmune diseases and nutrient malabsorption, to understand how these complex connections affect our digestion.

In addition, we will discover the importance of maintaining a healthy microbiota and how our diet and lifestyle habits can influence its balance. We will learn about the foods recommended to promote a healthy microbiota and how a personalized diet can be key to preventing the recurrence of SIBO and improving our digestive health.

Throughout this book, we will demystify scientific concepts and medical terms so you can easily understand how your digestive system works and how you can effectively care for it.

Our goal is to empower you with the knowledge and tools you need to make informed decisions about your digestive health. With the right support and guidance from health professionals, you will be able to effectively address SIBO and other digestive conditions, and cultivate a healthy microbiota that gives you a full and vital life.

It is important to note that these risk factors do not necessarily directly cause SIBO, but they can increase the likelihood of developing it. In addition, some people may have more than one risk factor that contributes to the onset of this disorder.

So get ready to embark on this exciting journey towards digestive balance, where we will discover how our health starts on the inside and how we can nourish our body and mind to achieve optimal health and wellness. Let us go together to explore the secrets of a healthy microbiota and discover the transformative power it can have on our lives!

WHAT IS SIBO?

DEFINITION AND CONCEPT

SIBO (Small Intestinal Bacterial Overgrowth) is a gastrointestinal disorder characterized by an abnormal and excessive increase of bacteria in the small intestine. Under normal conditions, the small intestine should contain a relatively low number of bacteria compared to the large intestine, as it is in this latter part of the digestive tract that bacterial fermentation and nutrient absorption mainly occur.

SIBO is not a new condition. Gastroenterologists have been aware of SIBO since the 1950s and 1960s when it was linked to problems with poor digestion or malabsorption. According to Dr. Santos, the concept of SIBO has evolved from being a complication associated with gastrointestinal surgery, intestinal motility disorders such as scleroderma or diabetes, or insufficient gastric juice production, to becoming an epidemic disorder present in otherwise healthy individuals. SIBO is also common in patients with symptoms similar to irritable bowel syndrome, as approximately 35% of them experience SIBO at some point in their lives.

Although the cause of intestinal bacterial overgrowth is not fully understood in all patients, any condition that blocks the intestine or slows it down can lead to SIBO. Food poisoning, for example, has recently been identified as a cause of slowed transit in the small intestine in studies with rats.

Medications that alter intestinal motility, such as antibiotics, opioids, and anticholinergics, can also promote bacterial overgrowth in some people. However, Dr. Santos mentioned that it is common for patients with SIBO to have unfounded fears about consuming gluten-containing foods and medications like omeprazole, as they believe these can cause SIBO, although this relationship has not been sufficiently proven.

In the case of SIBO, bacteria normally found in the colon move into the small intestine and begin to multiply excessively. This uncontrolled proliferation of bacteria can lead to impaired digestive function and inadequate absorption of nutrients, as the bacteria may consume some of the nutrients before the body has a chance to absorb them properly.

Bacteria present in the small intestine can produce gas and toxic substances, which can lead to uncomfortable gastrointestinal symptoms and various health problems. These symptoms can vary significantly from person to person, but some of the most common include:

- Abdominal bloating

- Excessive flatulence (gas)

- Diarrhea (diarrhea)

- Constipation

- Abdominal pain and cramping

- Bloating after eating

- General discomfort

It is important to note that SIBO is not a single disease in itself, but rather a syndrome associated with a number of underlying conditions that can affect the normal function of the small intestine. Among the conditions that may predispose to SIBO are alterations in intestinal motility (movement of food through the digestive tract), physical obstructions, prolonged use of certain medications, problems in the immune system, among others.

The diagnosis of SIBO is made through different tests, such as the exhaled hydrogen test and the exhaled methane test, which measure the gases produced by bacteria during the fermentation of carbohydrates in the small intestine.

Treatment of SIBO usually involves a combination of approaches, which may include the use of specific antibiotics to eliminate excess bacteria, dietary changes to reduce fermentation and promote a healthier intestinal environment, and management of underlying conditions that may be contributing to SIBO.

It is essential to adequately address SIBO because, if left untreated, it can lead to long-term complications, such as malabsorption of essential nutrients, nutritional deficiencies, and an overall deterioration in the patient's quality of life. Therefore, it is crucial that individuals experiencing symptoms related to SIBO seek medical attention and undergo the necessary tests for accurate diagnosis and effective treatment.

CAUSES OF SIBO

SIBO (Small Intestinal Bacterial Overgrowth) can have a variety of causes, and in many cases, results from a combination of factors that contribute to an imbalance in the gut microbiota. The following are some of the most common causes that can lead to the development of SIBO:

Proper movement of food contents through the digestive tract is crucial to prevent stagnation and bacterial buildup in the small intestine. If the functioning of the muscles and nerves responsible for peristalsis (the contractile movements that propel contents through the digestive system) is compromised, bacteria are more likely to become trapped and multiply excessively.

Any condition that causes narrowing or blockage of the small intestine can lead to a buildup of bacteria in that area. This could be the result of adhesions, scarring, hernias, or tumors that interfere with the normal flow of contents through the intestine.

The pH of the small intestine is a crucial factor in maintaining the balance of bacteria. If the pH becomes less acidic than normal, it can encourage the overgrowth of certain types of bacteria normally found in the colon.

A weakened immune system may not be able to adequately control bacterial growth in the small intestine, which may allow bacteria to proliferate unchecked.

Surgical interventions in the abdomen can alter intestinal anatomy and motility, which increases the risk of developing SIBO.

Prolonged use of certain medications, such as proton pump inhibitors (PPIs) and broad-spectrum antibiotics, can alter the composition of the intestinal microbiota and promote bacterial overgrowth in the small intestine.

In some cases, SIBO may be related to congenital malformations affecting the development of the intestine.

Certain gastrointestinal conditions, such as Crohn's disease, celiac disease, diverticulitis, and other inflammatory bowel diseases, may increase the risk of SIBO due to altered intestinal environment and motility.

In some people, SIBO may develop after exposure to harmful bacteria in water or food while traveling or living in areas with poor hygienic conditions.

Importantly, in some cases, the exact cause of SIBO can be difficult to determine, and may be the result of a combination of multiple factors. A proper diagnosis and a comprehensive approach to treating SIBO can help address the underlying causes and improve the patient's symptoms and quality of life.

RISK FACTORS

People with compromised immune systems, such as those with HIV/AIDS, cancer or who have received immunosuppressive treatments, may be at increased risk for SIBO due to the immune system's inability to control bacterial growth. Older people may have an increased risk of SIBO due to natural changes in the digestive system and an increased likelihood of chronic medical conditions.

International travel or exposure to contaminated food and water: In some cases, SIBO may develop after exposure to harmful bacteria in food or water while traveling or living in areas with poor hygiene conditions.

SIBO SYMPTOMS AND DIAGNOSIS

COMMON SYMPTOMS OF SIBO

Symptoms of SIBO (Small Intestinal Bacterial Overgrowth) can vary in severity and present differently in each individual. Some people may experience mild symptoms, while others may experience more significant discomfort. Common symptoms of SIBO include:

Abdominal distension: It is one of the most characteristic symptoms of SIBO. People may feel that their abdomen is swollen or inflamed, which can lead to a feeling of having a "swollen belly" even after eating small portions of food.

Excessive flatulence (gas): Bacterial overgrowth in the small intestine can lead to an increased amount of gas, which can lead to an increased frequency of belching and flatulence.

Diarrhea: Some people with SIBO may experience diarrhea, which may be watery and of variable frequency. Diarrhea results from excessive food-fermenting bacteria in the small intestine, leading to the production of waste products and gases.

Constipation: Although it may seem contradictory, constipation can also be a symptom of SIBO. Bacterial overgrowth can interfere with proper movement of the small intestine, leading to slower bowel movement and stool accumulation.

Abdominal pain and cramping: Excessive bacteria can cause irritation and inflammation in the small intestine, which can cause abdominal pain, cramping, and a general feeling of illness (malaise).

Swelling after eating: People with SIBO may notice a significant increase in abdominal swelling after meals, especially if they have eaten foods rich in fermentable carbohydrates.

Malaise: SIBO can impair proper absorption of nutrients, which can lead to nutritional deficiencies and general malaise. People may feel weak, fatigued, or experience unintentional weight loss.

Extraintestinal symptoms: Some people with SIBO may have symptoms outside the gastrointestinal tract, such as joint pains, headaches, skin problems, chronic fatigue, or neurologic problems, which may be related to systemic inflammation caused by bacterial overgrowth.

DIFFERENCES BETWEEN SIBO AND OTHER GASTROINTESTINAL DISORDERS

It is important to understand the differences between SIBO (Small Intestine Bacterial Overgrowth) and other gastrointestinal disorders, as many of them may have similar symptoms but require different diagnostic and treatment approaches.

In the following chapters we will see the details of the differences between each one. Meanwhile, here are some key differences between SIBO and other common gastrointestinal disorders:

SIBO vs. Irritable Bowel Syndrome (SIBO):

SIBO is characterized by an overgrowth of bacteria in the small intestine, while SIBO is a functional bowel disorder that manifests with symptoms

Treatment of SIBO in people with IBD may be needed to relieve additional symptoms caused by bacterial overgrowth, but the main treatment focuses on controlling inflammation with specific drugs.

SIBO vs. Gastresophageal Reflux Disease (GERD):

GERD is a condition in which stomach contents return to the esophagus, causing heartburn and burning in the chest.

Although gastrointestinal symptoms such as abdominal distention may be present in both conditions, SIBO focuses primarily on the small intestine, whereas GERD involves the esophagus and stomach.

Symptoms of GERD may improve with dietary changes and drugs to reduce stomach acidity, whereas SIBO requires specific treatments to control bacterial growth in the small intestine.

DIAGNOSTIC METHODS

Proper diagnosis of SIBO (Small Intestinal Bacterial Overgrowth) is essential to ensure effective treatment aimed at addressing small intestinal bacterial overgrowth. The main diagnostic methods used to detect SIBO are described below:

Lactulose Breath Test: This is one of the most common tests for SIBO diagnosis. During this test, the person swallows a solution of lactulose, a type of sugar that is not absorbed from the small intestine. If bacterial overgrowth occurs, the bacteria will break down lactulose, producing gases such as hydrogen and methane. These gases are detected and measured in the patient's breath at specific time intervals after ingesting lactulose. The presence of high concentrations of hydrogen and/or methane in the breath may suggest the presence of SIBO.

Glucose breath test: Similar to the lactulose test, but instead of lactulose, the patient swallows a glucose solution. Bacterial glucose fermentation also produces gases that can be detected and measured in breath to determine whether SIBO is present.

Duodenal fluid aspiration: In this procedure, an endoscope is passed through the mouth into the small intestine to obtain a sample of duodenal fluid. The sample is then tested for an elevated bacterial count, which could confirm the diagnosis of SIBO.

Culture of duodenal aspirate: Duodenal aspirate can also be used to grow (culture) the bacteria in the small intestine and evaluate the growth and types of bacteria in it. This approach can provide valuable information about the type of bacteria present and their susceptibility to antibiotics.

Lactose or fructose breath test: Some practitioners may also use lactose or fructose-specific breath tests because these substances are susceptible to fermentation by bacteria in the small intestine. These tests can help identify food intolerances and the bacterial overgrowth associated with these intolerances.

It is essential that these tests are performed and evaluated by health professionals trained in the diagnosis and treatment of SIBO, since the interpretation of the results can be complex and treatment must be personalized for each individual. With proper diagnosis, a treatment plan can be established that includes dietary changes, specific antibiotics, and/or natural approaches to control and prevent small-bowel bacterial overgrowth and improve the patient's quality of life.

CONTRIBUTING FACTORS
TO SIBO DEVELOPMENT

INTESTINAL MOTOR DYSFUNCTION

Intestinal motor dysfunction is one of the most important contributing factors in the development of SIBO (Small Intestinal Bacterial Overgrowth). Proper movement of the contents through the gastrointestinal tract is essential for proper digestion and absorption of nutrients as well as preventing the stagnation of bacteria in the small intestine.

When intestinal motility is compromised, different conditions that favor bacterial overgrowth can occur:

Hypomotility: A decrease in the activity of the muscles and nerves responsible for peristalsis (rhythmic, coordinated movement of the gastrointestinal tract) can cause slow intestinal transit. This means that food and digestive juices stay longer in the small intestine, allowing more time for bacteria to multiply and creating an environment conducive to their proliferation.

Intestinal stasis: Intestinal stasis refers to the stagnation or accumulation of content in the small intestine due to decreased motility. This accumulation of undigested material and bacteria can create a suitable environment for excessive growth of bacteria.

Motor migration is a coordinated pattern of movement in the small intestine between meals that helps eliminate bacteria and debris. When motor migration is impaired, these natural cleanings are not done, which can lead to bacteria retention.

Intestinal stenosis or narrowing: Any blockage or narrowing in the small intestine can block the normal passage of food and fluids, causing bacteria to accumulate in the upper part of the small intestine.

Neuromuscular disorders: Certain neuromuscular conditions, such as scleroderma, diabetes, irritable bowel syndrome, and Parkinson disease, can affect the motor function of the intestine and increase the risk of SIBO.

Previous abdominal surgeries: Abdominal surgeries can cause adhesions and changes in anatomy, which can alter intestinal motility and contribute to the development of SIBO.

Intestinal motor dysfunction may occur as an isolated factor or may be part of a broader medical condition. It is important to address this dysfunction, as it may be one of the underlying causes of SIBO and significantly affect patients' quality of life. Effective SIBO treatment should include approaches that address bowel motility, such as dietary changes, prokinetic drugs (which stimulate bowel movement), and lifestyle approaches that promote healthy bowel function.

STRUCTURAL PROBLEMS AND OBSTRUCTIONS

Structural problems and small-bowel obstructions may be crucial factors contributing to the development of SIBO (Small-Bowel Bacterial Overgrowth). These conditions can cause an alteration in the normal flow of food and fluids through the small intestine, creating an environment conducive to the overgrowth of bacteria. Some of the specific factors related to structural problems and obstructions that may contribute to SIBO are described below:

Abdominal adhesions: Adhesions are bands of scar tissue that form in the abdomen after surgery, inflammation, or injury. These adhesions can join different small-bowel structures, causing partial narrowing or blockage that makes the normal passage of intestinal contents difficult. Bacteria may become trapped in these areas and multiply excessively, resulting in SIBO.

Intestinal scarring: Certain conditions or surgeries can leave scars in the small intestine, which can lead to a reduction in the diameter of the intestinal lumen. This can lead to a narrowing of the intestine and, in turn, a partial blockage that favors the accumulation of bacteria.

Intestinal hernias: A hernia occurs when a portion of the intestine protrudes through a weakness in the abdominal wall. This can lead to a partial strangulation or blockage of the intestine, which favors the development of SIBO in that region.

Tumors and intestinal polyps: Tumors or polyps that develop in the small intestine can cause blockages or narrowing that prevent the proper passage of intestinal contents.

Congenital stenosis: Some people may be born with congenital anatomic narrowing in the small intestine, which may predispose to SIBO.

Diverticula of the intestine: Diverticula are small sacs or pouches that can form in the wall of the small intestine. These pockets can trap intestinal contents, allowing bacteria to accumulate and multiply in the area.

Importantly, not all people with structural problems or blockages in the small intestine will develop SIBO. However, these conditions may increase the risk of bacterial overgrowth due to disruption of normal flow of intestinal contents and creation of pockets or stagnant areas.

Managing these structural problems may involve addressing the underlying conditions using surgery or endoscopic procedures, to improve bowel flow and reduce the risk of SIBO. In some cases, SIBO may be recurrent if underlying structural problems are not adequately addressed.

IMMUNE SYSTEM DISORDERS

Immune system disorders may also be contributing factors to the development of SIBO (Small Intestine Bacterial Overgrowth). The immune system plays a crucial role in controlling and regulating the gut microbiota, helping to maintain an appropriate balance between beneficial and potentially harmful bacteria. When the immune system is compromised or dysfunctional, there may be a loss of the ability to control bacterial growth in the small intestine, facilitating the development of SIBO. The following are specific situations related to immune system disorders that may increase the risk of SIBO:

Primary immunodeficiencies: Primary immunodeficiencies are genetic disorders in which the immune system malfunctions because of defects in the genes responsible for its function. These defects can affect the production of immune cells or the ability of these cells to recognize and kill harmful bacteria. People with primary immunodeficiencies may be more susceptible to bacterial overgrowth in the small intestine.

Acquired immunodeficiencies: Certain conditions and diseases, such as HIV/AIDS and cancer, can weaken the immune system, which can lead to increased bacterial proliferation in the small intestine.

Autoimmune diseases: Some autoimmune diseases, such as Sjögren's syndrome, Crohn's disease, and ulcerative colitis, involve an overactive immune response that can affect the gut microbiota and increase the risk of SIBO.

Use of immunosuppressive drugs: Immunosuppressive drugs, such as corticosteroids and some chemotherapeutic agents, are used to treat various conditions, but they can also weaken the immune system and increase susceptibility to SIBO.

Deregulation of the local immune response: In the small intestine, the immune system plays a key role in controlling bacterial growth. Decreased local immune response in the intestine may allow bacteria to multiply excessively.

Management of immune system disorders can vary depending on the specific condition and severity of the immune involvement. In some cases, the use of immunomodulatory medicinal products may be necessary to improve immune function and reduce the risk of SIBO. However, any treatment should be managed and supervised by a health care practitioner specialized in immunology or gastroenterology to ensure appropriate and personalized care.

RELATED UNDERLYING CONDITIONS

Related underlying diseases are key factors that can contribute to the development of SIBO (Small Intestine Bacterial Overgrowth). Some medical conditions can alter the intestinal environment and motor function of the intestine, making it easier for bacteria to grow too much in the small intestine. Some of the underlying diseases that are associated with an increased risk of SIBO are described below:

Crohn' s disease:

Crohn's disease emerges as a complex medical challenge, highlighting its chronic inflammatory intestinal nature that can unfold in any segment of the extensive gastrointestinal tract. My experience of more than two decades in the medical field has allowed me to understand in depth the interrelations between this pathology and the SIBO, providing an integral perspective for those who seek clarification on these issues.

At the heart of Crohn disease lies persistent inflammation that, unfortunately, leads to alterations in the intestinal anatomy. This inflammatory process not only impacts the structural integrity of the intestine, but also triggers motor dysfunction that, in turn, can contribute to such as abdominal pain, swelling, and changes in bowel habits without evidence of structural damage or inflammation.

Although some symptoms may overlap, SIBO often causes more pronounced abdominal swelling and distention due to excessive gas production by bacteria in the small intestine.

The diagnosis of SIBO is based primarily on presenting symptoms and excluding other conditions, whereas SIBO is confirmed by specific breath tests to measure bacterial gas production.

SIBO vs. Celiac disease:

Celiac disease is an autoimmune disease in which gluten (a protein found in wheat, barley, and rye) triggers an inflammatory reaction in the small intestine.

Although celiac disease can cause gastrointestinal symptoms similar to SIBO, such as diarrhea, bloating, and pain, the underlying cause is different, and treatment involves eliminating gluten from the diet.

People with SIBO may experience improved or resolved symptoms when treating bacterial overgrowth, while people with celiac disease need to maintain a gluten-free diet for life.

IBD vs. Inflammatory Bowel Diseases (IBD):

IBDs, such as Crohn disease and ulcerative colitis, are chronic autoimmune disorders that cause inflammation in the gastrointestinal tract.

Although some people with IBD may have IBD as a secondary complication due to motor dysfunction or alterations in the gut microbiota, the presence of IBD is mainly characterized by inflammation and structural damage of the gut.

the development of SIBO. The interaction between these two conditions should not be underestimated, since chronic inflammation compromises the ability of the intestine to perform its functions properly, predisposing the patient to increased susceptibility to bacterial overgrowth.

The similarities and synergies between Crohn's disease and SIBO are clinically revealing. Both entities share an inflammatory background, creating a breeding ground for uncontrolled bacterial overgrowth in the small intestine. This phenomenon, which I frequently observe in my clinical practice, underscores the importance of comprehensively addressing both the underlying inflammation of Crohn's disease and the resulting SIBO.

But it is crucial to recognize the differences between these conditions. While Crohn's disease manifests primarily as an inflammatory disease, SIBO is characterized by bacterial overgrowth in the upper gastrointestinal tract. My therapeutic approach has been shaped by years of experience in managing patients with these conditions, allowing me to discern between the specific challenges associated with each one.

Ulcerative colitis:

Ulcerative colitis, a medical condition that shares the category of inflammatory bowel diseases, stands as a topic of special interest in my extensive career of more than two decades in the field of medicine and therapies. Although its primary impact is manifested in the colon and rectum, it is imperative to highlight the complexity of this condition, since some individuals experience an extension of the inflammatory process to the small intestine, generating an intriguing connection with bacterial overgrowth syndrome (BOS).

My clinical experience has witnessed the variability in the presentation of ulcerative colitis, a fact that often surprises patients and colleagues alike. Those affected by this disease may exhibit not only the typical inflammation in the colon, but also a spread to the small intestine. This peculiarity, although not a universal feature of ulcerative colitis, opens an enlightening dialog on the intersections between this pathology and SIBO.

Simply put, ulcerative colitis and SIBO share a potentially convergent predisposition when inflammation spreads beyond its primary location. Persistent inflammation in the small intestine, as a result of the spread of ulcerative colitis, can create an environment conducive to the development of SIBO. This relationship is essential to understand the complexities associated with managing patients who face both conditions simultaneously.

While the former is characterized by chronic inflammation in the colon and rectum, SIBO is distinguished by bacterial overgrowth in the small intestine. This distinction has a direct impact on the therapeutic strategies that I use in my daily practice, where the personalization of approaches is essential to address the specific needs of each patient.

Celiac disease:

Celiac disease, a medical entity that has captured my attention and expertise over two decades in the field of medicine and therapies, represents a telling example of the interrelationship between autoimmune conditions and bacterial overgrowth syndrome (BIS). Its autoimmune origin, triggered by exposure to gluten in wheat, barley, and rye, places celiac disease in a distinct niche of pathologies that share similarities and significant connections with SIBO.

In my clinical experience, I have observed how the chronic intestinal inflammation characteristic of celiac disease not only confines its effects to the immune system, but also influences the motor function of the small intestine. This crucial connection between persistent inflammation and motor dysfunction creates an enabling environment for the development of SIBO. The complex interaction between these two conditions demands an insightful and personalized clinical approach, highlighting the need for a deep understanding of the complexities involved.

It is essential to note that celiac disease and SIBO share a potentially convergent pathway: impaired small-bowel motor function. The chronic inflammation characteristic of celiac disease, triggered by the autoimmune response to gluten, can compromise the ability of the small intestine to perform its functions efficiently, predisposing the individual to an increased risk of SIBO.

Despite these similarities, differences between celiac disease and SIBO are critical to effective management. While the former is an autoimmune disease triggered by gluten intolerance, SIBO is distinguished by bacterial overgrowth in the small intestine. My more than two decades of experience have consolidated my focus on therapeutic strategies that address both celiac disease and SIBO, recognizing the importance of personalizing treatment to meet the specific needs of each patient.

Diverticulosis:

This condition, characterized by the formation of small bags or sacs in the wall of the colon, poses an intriguing clinical picture that, in some cases, is intertwined surprisingly with the development of SIBO.

In my practice, I have treated patients with diverticulosis and have observed how this condition can evolve into diverticulitis, a state in which the bursae become inflamed or infected. However, beyond these recognized manifestations, my experience has revealed an underlying connection between diverticulosis and SIBO, highlighting the importance of a holistic understanding in managing these conditions.

Diverticulosis, by affecting the anatomy of the colon, can create favorable ground for SIBO. The formation of these small pockets not only alters the structure of the large intestine but can also influence the dynamics of the small intestine. The interrelation between these two conditions highlights the need for a comprehensive evaluation that considers both structural and functional factors in the search for an effective therapeutic approach.

Diverticulosis involves pockets forming in the colon, SIBO is characterized by bacterial overgrowth in the small intestine. My professional approach thrives on understanding these differences, enabling me to design specific therapeutic strategies that address each patient's unique needs.

Irritable bowel syndrome (SIBO):

Irritable Bowel Syndrome (SIBO) represents a multifaceted clinical challenge that, throughout my more than 20 years of experience in medicine and therapies, has aroused a deep interest and attention in my practice. Although the precise cause of SIBO remains largely elusive, it is postulated that changes in intestinal motility and alterations in the microbiota play a crucial role in its manifestation. This intriguing overview leads us to explore the connections between SIBO and bacterial overgrowth syndrome (BIS), highlighting fundamental similarities and differences.

In my career as a health professional, I have observed how alterations in intestinal motility, characterized by changes in the contraction and relaxation of intestinal muscles, can predispose certain individuals to develop SIBO in the context of SIBO. The relationship between these two syndromes reveals the complexity of intestinal interactions and highlights the importance of a comprehensive approach to address these concurrent conditions.

Intestinal microbiota, a diverse community of microorganisms that inhabit our digestive tract, also emerges as a key player in the SIBO equation and its potential connection to SIBO. It has been suggested that imbalances in bacterial composition may contribute to SIBO symptomatology and, in some cases, lead to bacterial overgrowth in the small intestine. This understanding sheds light on the importance of considering not only the symptoms of SIBO, but also the possible complications, such as SIBO, which may arise as a result of these alterations.

SIBO manifests as a set of gastrointestinal symptoms, SIBO is specifically characterized by bacterial overgrowth in the small intestine. My clinical approach is based on this precise understanding, allowing me to design therapeutic strategies aimed at the specific needs of each patient.

Pancreatic dysfunctions:

The insufficient production of pancreatic enzymes emerges as a critical element that can trigger a cascade of events harmful to the digestion and absorption of nutrients, providing an enlightening perspective on the relationship between these conditions.

The main function of pancreatic enzymes is to break down food into simpler components, thus facilitating its absorption in the small intestine. When the production of these enzymes is compromised, either due to underlying medical conditions or physiological factors, an imbalance in the digestive process is triggered. This mismatch not only affects the breakdown of food, but may also lead to an environment conducive to bacterial growth in the small intestine.

The connection between inadequate production of pancreatic enzymes and SIBO lies in disruption of the protective barrier of the small intestine. Insufficient pancreatic enzymes can result in inefficient digestion, generating non-decomposed food residues that act as an ideal substrate for bacterial overgrowth. This phenomenon, observed in clinical practice, highlights the importance of addressing not only the symptoms of SIBO, but also the underlying causes that can trigger or perpetuate this bacterial imbalance.

Despite the similarities in the pathophysiological field, it is essential to distinguish the differences between insufficient pancreatic enzyme production and SIBO. While the first focuses on enzyme dysfunction and its impact on digestion, SIBO is characterized by abnormal bacterial growth in the small intestine. My clinical approach is based on this differentiated understanding, allowing me to address each aspect in a specific and effective way.

Blind loop syndrome:

In the vast panoply of diseases related to Bacterial Overgrowth Syndrome (BIS), the presence of a blind loop or deviation of a part of the small intestine represents a particularly intriguing medical entity. This condition, which may arise for a variety of reasons, creates an enabling environment for SIBO by facilitating the accumulation of intestinal contents. Over the course of my two-decade career in medicine and therapeutics, I have deepened my understanding of this phenomenon and its interconnectedness with bacterial overgrowth.

Creating a blind loop, or diverting a portion of the small intestine, lays the groundwork for a number of gastrointestinal challenges. This isolated segment can become a reservoir where intestinal contents accumulate, providing fertile ground for abnormal bacterial development. In my clinical practice, I have observed how this anatomical configuration can predispose patients to SIBO, underlining the importance of a comprehensive evaluation in the management of these conditions.

The similarity between the formation of a blind loop and SIBO lies in the creation of an environment conducive to bacterial growth in the small intestine. In both cases, the accumulation of intestinal contents acts as a catalyst for the proliferation of bacteria, generating a series of gastrointestinal symptoms that require specialized attention and management.

But it is imperative to highlight the crucial differences between these conditions. While SIBO is specifically characterized by bacterial overgrowth in the small intestine, the formation of a blind loop focuses on the anatomy of the intestine, creating a reservoir where the bacteria can thrive. My therapeutic approach is based on this distinction, as I seek to address the underlying causes and specific manifestations of each condition precisely.

SIBO TREATMENTS

SIBO TREATMENTS ANTIBIOTICS AND PROBIOTICS

Treatment of SIBO (Small-Bowel Bacterial Overgrowth) may involve multifaceted approaches to address bacterial overgrowth and relieve associated symptoms. The most common treatments for SIBO include the use of antibiotics and probiotics. Both approaches are explained below:

Antibiotics: Antibiotics are the cornerstone of SIBO treatment, as they are used to reduce and control the overgrowth of bacteria in the small intestine. Specific antibiotics used for SIBO include:

Rifaximin: It is a non-absorbable antibiotic that targets bacteria in the small intestine. It is the treatment of choice for SIBO because of its effectiveness and safety. Rifaximin acts locally in the intestine without significantly affecting the intestinal microbiota of the colon. It is usually given over a course of two weeks or more, depending on the severity of the SIBO.

Neomycin: Another antibiotic used in the treatment of SIBO. It is often combined with rifaximin to increase the effectiveness of treatment. Neomycin may have more effects on the gut microbiota and is usually used in combination with rifaximin only when methane-containing bacterial overgrowth (M-SIBO) is suspected.

Ciprofloxacin: In some cases, when rifaximin is not available or not effective, ciprofloxacin can be used as an alternative. However, its use may be limited due to bacterial resistance and its effects on the gut microbiota.

It is important that the choice and duration of antibiotic treatment is determined by a healthcare professional experienced in the treatment of SIBO. After antibiotic treatment, doctors often recommend approaches to restoring the health of the gut microbiota, such as using probiotics.

Probiotics: Probiotics are beneficial living organisms that can be found in certain foods and supplements. After antibiotic treatment, the intestinal microbiota may be altered, which may adversely affect gastrointestinal health. Probiotics can help restore the balance of the microbiota and support gut health.

Lactobacillus: This genus of probiotic bacteria is one of the most studied and has been widely used to support gastrointestinal health.

Bifidobacterium: Another genus of common probiotic bacteria that can benefit intestinal health.

Saccharomyces boulardii: This is a yeast probiotic that may be beneficial for certain people with SIBO and can help prevent bacterial overgrowth from recurring.

It is important to note that not all probiotics are suitable for all people with SIBO, as individual response may vary. Some people may experience significant improvement with probiotics, whereas others may have increased sensitivity and need to adjust the dose or type of probiotic used.

CHANGES IN DIET

Here we will see, in a simple and essential way, the changes that are advisable in our diet. It will be in the next chapter that, at the risk of repeating some concepts, the dietary aspect for SIBO is further developed.

Dietary and dietary changes are a key component in the treatment of SIBO (Small Intestinal Bacterial Overgrowth). Diet plays a crucial role in regulating the gut microbiota and can help reduce bacterial overgrowth in the small intestine. Here are some common dietary approaches used in the treatment of SIBO:

Low-fermentable carbohydrate diet: Fermentable carbohydrates are those that are difficult to digest and absorb in the small intestine and are thus fermented by bacteria, which produces gases and can promote SIBO. A low-fermentable carbohydrate diet, known as the FODMAP (Fermentable Oligosaccharides, Disaccharides, Monosaccharides, and Polyols) diet, restricts certain FODMAP-rich foods to reduce the fermentative load on the intestine. Some of the restricted foods in this diet include certain fruits, vegetables, dairy products, legumes, and artificial sweeteners.

Specific carbohydrate diet: Some people with SIBO may benefit from a specific carbohydrate diet (SCD) or a limited fermentable carbohydrate diet (LOFFLEX) that also restricts certain fermentable carbohydrates to reduce the bacterial load in the small intestine.

Intermittent fasting, under the supervision of a health care practitioner, can help decrease the bacterial population in the small intestine by providing periods of digestive rest.

Instead of eating large meals, it may be helpful to divide meals into smaller portions and distribute them throughout the day. This can reduce the burden on the digestive system and improve intestinal motility.

Each person with SIBO may have specific foods that trigger or exacerbate their symptoms. Identifying and avoiding these foods can help improve quality of life and reduce inflammation and irritation in the intestine.

It is important to mention that the choice of diet may vary depending on the severity of the SIBO, individual symptoms, and personal preferences. In addition, it is essential that any dietary modification be performed under the supervision and guidance of a health professional, especially a dietitian or nutritionist specialized in gastrointestinal disorders.

Dietary SIBO treatment is generally combined with other approaches, such as the use of antibiotics or probiotics, to address all aspects of bacterial overgrowth and promote the restoration of intestinal health. A comprehensive and personalized approach is essential for the effective management of SIBO and to improve the quality of life of the patient.

NATURAL AND COMPLEMENTARY APPROACHES

Natural and complementary approaches may also play a role in the treatment of SIBO (Small Intestinal Bacterial Overgrowth), especially as part of an integrative and multifaceted approach. While these approaches alone may not be sufficient to treat SIBO, they can complement other treatments and help improve bowel symptoms and health. Some natural and complementary approaches that have been investigated and used in the treatment of SIBO are described below:

Essential oils: Some essential oils, such as oregano oil, peppermint oil and cinnamon oil, have shown antimicrobial properties and can help reduce bacterial growth in the small intestine. They can be taken as capsules or diluted in carrier oil for topical use.

Phytotherapy: Some herbs and medicinal plants have antimicrobial and anti-inflammatory properties that can help control bacterial growth in the small intestine and relieve symptoms of SIBO. Some herbs used in this context include berberine, garlic, ursi grapes, thyme, and echinacea.

Natural Prokinetics: Prokinetics are drugs that improve intestinal motility and can help prevent the stagnation of bacteria in the small intestine. Some natural approaches such as ginger, Chinese ginger (ginseng), licorice root, and acupuncture have been used to stimulate gastrointestinal motility and improve bowel function.

Digestive enzymes: Digestive enzymes can help improve digestion and absorption of nutrients, which can reduce the availability of substrates for bacterial growth in the small intestine. Digestive enzyme supplementation may be helpful for some people with SIBO.

Immune modulation therapies: Some immune modulation therapies, such as immunotherapy, can help improve immune function and reduce inflammation in the intestine, which may be beneficial in people with immune-related SIBO.

It is essential to note that natural and complementary approaches to the treatment of SIBO must be used under the supervision of a trained health professional, as their effectiveness and safety may vary depending on the individual situation of each patient. In addition, it is important to remember that these approaches should not replace conventional treatments, such as the use of antibiotics or probiotics, which have been shown to be effective in the management of SIBO.

RECOMMENDATIONS FOR LONG-TERM MANAGEMENT

Long-term management of SIBO (Small Intestine Bacterial Overgrowth) is essential to prevent recurrence of symptoms and maintain good intestinal health. Once SIBO has been treated and symptoms have improved, it is important to implement strategies to reduce the risk of relapse. Here are some recommendations for the long-term management of SIBO:

Working with a dietitian or nutritionist who specializes in gastrointestinal disorders can help create a balanced, personalized diet that meets individual nutritional needs and reduces the fermentation burden on the small intestine. It is important to maintain an adequate balance of nutrients and avoid foods that may trigger SIBO symptoms.

Probiotics may be beneficial in restoring the health of the gut microbiota after treatment with antibiotics. However, choosing appropriate probiotics and following the recommendations of a health care practitioner are essential because some probiotics may not be suitable for all people with SIBO.

Stress can affect gastrointestinal function and intestinal motility, so it is important to implement strategies to manage stress, such as meditation, yoga, cognitive-behavioral therapy, and regular exercise.

Overuse of antibiotics may adversely affect the gut microbiota and increase the risk of SIBO recurrence. It is important to use antibiotics only when needed and under the supervision of a health care practitioner.

If SIBO is related to an underlying disease, such as autoimmune diseases or immune system disorders, it is essential to adequately address and treat these conditions to reduce the risk of recurrence of SIBO.

Learning about SIBO and its triggers can help people make informed choices about their diet and lifestyle. Self-care, such as keeping track of symptoms and responses to certain foods, may be helpful in identifying patterns and triggers.

DIET BASICS FOR SIBO

Dietary fundamentals for SIBO focus on two key principles: limiting intake of sugars and starches and prioritizing low-FODMAP foods. This dietary approach is designed to reduce bacterial fermentation in the small intestine, which is the core of the problem at SIBO.

LIMITING SUGARS AND STARCHES

Dietary modification plays a critical role in the management of small-bowel bacterial overgrowth (SIBO), and a key aspect of this modification is sugar and starch limitation. Simple sugars and starches, which are found abundantly in many processed and refined foods, such as white breads, cakes, biscuits, and sugary drinks, are fermentable and can be rapidly used by abnormal bacteria in the small intestine. This fermentation produces gases and compounds that can cause symptoms such as swelling, pain, and alterations in the intestinal transit, characteristics of SIBO.

The increasing presence of sugars in a normal diet is a phenomenon that reflects changes in the patterns of food consumption and practices of the food industry over the last decades. This increase is partly due to the industrialization of food, where added sugars are often used to improve the taste, texture, and shelf life of products. Sugars are found not only in sweet foods and beverages, but also in less obvious products such as sauces, salad dressings, breads, processed meat products, and precooked foods. This fact contributes to an inadvertent increase in sugar consumption in the daily diet.

The pervasiveness of sugar in the modern diet poses several public health problems, including an increase in the prevalence of obesity, type 2 diabetes, cardiovascular disease, and other diet-related conditions. Sugars, especially when consumed in substantial amounts, can cause spikes in blood glucose levels and, in the long term, lead to insulin resistance, increasing the risk of metabolic diseases.

Being aware of what we eat means understanding and recognizing the presence of added sugars in our diet and making informed decisions about our dietary intake. This includes reading carefully the labels of food products, where added sugars can appear under numerous names, such as sucrose, fructose, dextrose, high fructose corn syrup, honey, maltose, and other terms that end in "-osa" or include the word "syrup".

Adopting conscious eating also means prioritizing whole, minimally processed foods over ultra-processed products. Foods such as fresh fruits, vegetables, whole grains, legumes, nuts, and seeds are naturally low in added sugars and provide a wide range of essential nutrients, including fibers, vitamins, and minerals, which are critical to maintaining health.

Restriction of sugars and starches aims to reduce the fermentation burden in the small intestine, thereby decreasing the growth and activity of pathogenic bacteria. By reducing the availability of these nutrients to bacteria, their proliferation and subsequent negative effects on gut health can be limited. Importantly, this restriction must be balanced to ensure that the body receives the energy and nutrients necessary for its optimal functioning. Sources of complex carbohydrates that are less fermentable and slower to digest, such as whole grains, should be selected to maintain energy and overall health.

Limiting sugars and starches should be part of a broader dietary approach that also includes adequate intake of healthy fibers, proteins, and fats to ensure complete nutrition. Fiber, in particular, should be consumed in adequate amounts and sourced from sources that are tolerable to the person with SIBO because some fibers can exacerbate symptoms in certain individuals. The right balance of nutrients helps promote normal intestinal motility and supports the health of the microbial ecosystem in the digestive tract.

Limiting dietary sugars and starches for SIBO is a key strategy that seeks to reduce the substrate available for fermentative bacteria in the small intestine, helping to control bacterial growth and relieve symptoms associated with SIBO. This strategy must be carefully implemented, within a comprehensive and personalized dietary plan, to ensure that all nutritional needs are met and long-term gut health is promoted.

PREFER LOW FODMAP FOODS

Low-FODMAP foods are foods that contain reduced levels of certain types of fermentable carbohydrates, which can cause digestive symptoms in some people, especially those with disorders such as irritable bowel syndrome (SIBO) or small-bowel bacterial overgrowth (SIBO). FODMAP is an acronym that represents:

Fermentable: Refers to the ability of microorganisms in the colon to break down (ferment) carbohydrates for use as an energy source.

Oligosaccharides: They include fructans and galactooligosaccharides (GOS) found in foods such as wheat, onion, garlic, and legumes.

Disaccharides: Mainly lactose, present in dairy products such as milk and cheese.

Monosaccharides: Essentially fructose, which is in greater quantity than glucose in certain fruits, such as apples and pears.

And:

Polyols: Sugar alcohols such as sorbitol and mannitol, found in some fruits and vegetables and also used as sweeteners.

Low-FODMAP diets focus on reducing consumption of these carbohydrates, which are poorly absorbed by the small intestine and can cause symptoms such as bloating, gas, abdominal pain, and bowel rhythm disturbances when fermented by intestinal bacteria. The idea is to minimize the load of these fermentable carbohydrates to relieve pressure on the digestive system.

Importantly, the low-FODMAP diet is not a permanent solution nor does it apply in the same way to all people. Initially, high-FODMAP food intake is reduced and then gradually reintroduced to identify specific foods that cause symptoms.

In the context of a low FODMAP diet, certain foods are identified that are generally well tolerated and can be consumed without causing the gastrointestinal symptoms associated with the malabsorption of these fermentable carbohydrates. Among these foods, we find a variety of fruits, such as bananas, blueberries, strawberries, and grapes. These fruits stand out for their lower FODMAP content compared to other fruits that may contain higher levels of fructose or polyols, making them safer choices for people sensitive to these carbohydrates.

In the field of vegetables, options such as carrots, peppers, spinach, and tomatoes are considered suitable for a diet low in FODMAP. These vegetables, besides being nutritious and rich in vitamins and minerals, have a low content of carbohydrates that can cause distention and discomfort in people with intolerance to FODMAP. Thus, including them in the diet helps maintain a balanced diet without sacrificing variety and taste.

As for protein, meat, fish, and eggs are naturally FODMAP-free, as these compounds are mainly found in carbohydrates and not in proteins. This means that these foods can be consumed without restrictions in terms of FODMAP content, which is beneficial for those who need to maintain adequate protein intake while managing their sensitivity to FODMAP.

Grains such as rice, quinoa, and oats are also generally well tolerated in a low-FODMAP diet. Although grains can be a source of carbohydrates, these specific options are low in FODMAP and thus less likely to cause symptoms.

They are an important source of energy and other essential nutrients, and their inclusion in the diet contributes to variety and satisfaction in meals.

Finally, in the dairy group, lactose-free alternatives, or vegetable milks such as almond milk are recommended for those who follow a diet low in FODMAP. These options prevent lactose, which is a disaccharide that some people cannot digest efficiently and can be a problem in high FODMAP diets. By choosing lactose-free or plant-based milk alternatives, you can enjoy the benefits of dairy products without the risks associated with lactose intolerance and SIBO symptoms.

In short, the selection of low-FODMAP foods involves opting for fruits, vegetables, protein, grains, and dairy that minimize the intake of fermentable carbohydrates. This dietary strategy allows people with sensitivity to these compounds to manage their symptoms effectively, while maintaining a nutritionally balanced and satisfying diet.

RECOMMENDED INGREDIENTS

In the SIBO diet, it is crucial to choose ingredients that are not only low in FODMAP but also promote gut health and general well-being. Vegetables play a primary role in this diet, with options such as spinach, carrots, eggplants, tomatoes, and courgettes standing out for their low FODMAP content. These vegetables are not only tolerable for people with SIBO, but also provide a wide range of essential nutrients, including vitamins, minerals, and fibers. For example, spinach and carrots are rich in vitamins A and C, while eggplants and courgettes offer a good source of fiber and antioxidants. The inclusion of these vegetables in the diet helps to ensure adequate nutrition and may contribute to improving bowel function.

As for proteins, it is essential for SIBO sufferers to include lean and easily digestible protein sources in their diet. Lean meats, fish, and eggs are excellent choices because they are high in quality protein and low in FODMAP, which helps prevent excessive bacterial fermentation in the small intestine. In addition, vegetable protein options like tofu and tempeh are valuable alternatives, especially for those who follow a vegetable diet or look for variety in their protein sources. These plant sources of protein are not only low in FODMAP but also contain other important nutrients, such as iron and calcium, and can be part of a balanced diet for SIBO management.

Low-FODMAP whole grains, such as quinoa, rice, and oats, are important components in a balanced SIBO diet. These grains provide complex carbohydrates, fibers, and a spectrum of essential vitamins and minerals, without causing the symptoms associated with SIBO. Quinoa, for example, is a whole grain that serves as an excellent source of whole proteins, while rice and oats are tolerated by most people with SIBO, offering a sustainable source of energy and being gentle in the digestive system.

Finally, healthy fats are a crucial element of a balanced diet and are especially important in managing SIBO. Olive oil, avocados, nuts, and seeds in moderation provide essential fatty acids and antioxidants that can help reduce inflammation and promote the overall health of the digestive system. In addition, these sources of healthy fats can improve the absorption of fat-soluble vitamins such as A, D, E, and K, thus contributing to optimal nutritional status.

An effective SIBO management diet should include a variety of low-FODMAP ingredients that together provide a full spectrum of nutrients needed for health maintenance. By properly combining vegetables, protein, whole grains and healthy fats, a balanced diet can be achieved that supports bowel function and improves the quality of life of people affected by SIBO.

.

BREAKFAST RECIPES

An option for breakfast could be a bowl of oats prepared with lactose-free milk or a vegetable alternative such as almond milk. Oats are a low-FODMAP whole grain and an excellent source of soluble fiber, which is beneficial for gut health. This dish can be supplemented with low-FODMAP fruits, such as strawberries or blueberries, and a pinch of cinnamon to add flavor without added sugars. For those who need an extra supply of protein, a handful of nuts or seeds can be added, considering that they should be consumed in moderation because of their fat content and FODMAPs.

For those who prefer a lighter dinner, especially if they experience more digestive symptoms at night, a large salad with a variety of vegetables low in FODMAP, such as spinach, tomatoes, cucumbers and an olive oil and lemon dressing, can be an excellent choice. Adding a source of lean protein, such as grilled chicken breast or tofu, can complete the meal, ensuring an adequate supply of nutrients without overloading the digestive system before sleep.

RELATIONSHIP BETWEEN SIBO
AND OTHER HEALTH CONDITIONS

S IBO (Small Intestinal Bacterial Overgrowth) is a gastrointestinal disorder increasingly recognized and studied in the field of medicine. It is characterized by an overgrowth of bacteria in the small intestine, which can lead to a series of digestive and systemic symptoms that significantly affect the quality of life of those who suffer from it. Although the SIBO is presented as a unique clinical entity, in recent years, increasing attention has been paid to its relationship with other health conditions.

This chapter aims to explore the close interaction between SIBO and other medical conditions, identifying how certain underlying diseases can predispose to or influence the development of bacterial overgrowth. Throughout these pages, we will examine in detail the relationship between SIBO and inflammatory bowel diseases, immune system disorders, intestinal motor dysfunctions, and other digestive and systemic conditions.

In this comprehensive analysis, we will examine the current scientific evidence supporting the association between SIBO and these health conditions. In addition, we will explore the underlying pathophysiological mechanisms that could explain how these diseases contribute to the development and persistence of bacterial overgrowth in the small intestine.

By understanding the relationship between SIBO and other health conditions, we will be able to take a more complete view of this complex clinical entity and move toward more comprehensive and personalized diagnostic and treatment approaches. Through the knowledge gained in this chapter, we hope to provide health professionals and patients with a solid foundation to effectively address SIBO and improve management of these concomitant health conditions.

SIBO AND IRRITABLE BOWEL SYNDROME (SIBO)

SIBO (Small Intestine Bacterial Overgrowth) and Irritable Bowel Syndrome (SIBO) are two common gastrointestinal disorders that often overlap and share similar symptoms, leading to increasing research into their relationship and possible association. Although they are different entities, it has been observed that a considerable proportion of people with SIBO also have SIBO, and vice versa. This overlap has led to the hypothesis that there is a bidirectional relationship between the two disorders.

SIBO is a chronic gastrointestinal tract disorder characterized by recurrent abdominal pain, abdominal distention, changes in bowel habits (diarrhea, constipation, or both), and pain relief after defecation. Although its exact cause is not fully understood, it is believed that factors such as altered intestinal motility, visceral hypersensitivity and alterations in the intestinal microbiota may contribute to the development of SIBO.

On the other hand, SIBO is a condition in which there is excessive growth of bacteria in the small intestine, where normally there should be a low bacterial population. SIBO can cause SIBO-like symptoms, such as abdominal distention, pain, and changes in bowel habits, leading to its association with SIBO.

Several studies have shown that a sizable proportion of people with SIBO also have SIBO, and it has been observed that successful treatment of SIBO may improve SIBO symptoms in some patients. However, the relationship between the two disorders is complex and not yet fully understood.

It has been proposed that SIBO could be a trigger or a contributing factor to the development of SIBO in some patients. Overgrowth of bacteria in the small intestine can impair intestinal motility and lead to increased visceral sensitivity, which would contribute to SIBO symptoms. On the other hand, some researchers suggest that certain alterations in intestinal motor function and visceral hypersensitivity associated with SIBO could predispose to the development of SIBO.

Treating SIBO in people with SIBO can be challenging, and a comprehensive approach is often taken that includes dietary changes, use of targeted antibiotics, and stress management. In addition, it has been observed that probiotics may be useful in some people with SIBO, although their use in the context of SIBO should be carefully considered, as certain probiotics could worsen bacterial overgrowth.

The relationship between SIBO and SIBO is an area of active and fascinating research in the field of gastroenterology. Although it has been shown that there is an overlap between both disorders, more research is needed to fully understand the nature of their association and how it can influence the therapeutic approach and clinical management of patients. It is important that health care practitioners consider this relationship in patients with chronic gastrointestinal symptoms and do more research to improve understanding and treatment of both disorders.

SIBO AND AUTOIMMUNE DISEASES

The relationship between SIBO (Small Intestine Bacterial Overgrowth) and autoimmune diseases is a growing research topic in the field of gastroenterology and immunology. An association between SIBO and certain autoimmune diseases has been observed, leading to the hypothesis that bacterial overgrowth in the small intestine could play a role in the development and/or exacerbation of these conditions.

Autoimmune diseases are disorders in which the body's immune system mistakenly attacks its own tissues and organs, causing inflammation and damage. Some of the autoimmune diseases that have been associated with SIBO include:

Celiac Disease: Celiac disease is an autoimmune disease triggered by the intake of gluten, a protein found in wheat, barley, and rye. Chronic inflammation and damage to the lining of the small intestine characteristic of celiac disease can impair intestinal motor function and increase the risk of SIBO.

Inflammatory Bowel Diseases (IBDs): Both Crohn's disease and ulcerative colitis, which are types of IBD, have been associated with an increased risk of IBD. Chronic inflammation and alteration of the intestinal microbiota under these conditions may contribute to the development of bacterial overgrowth in the small intestine.

Rheumatoid Arthritis: Rheumatoid arthritis is an autoimmune disease that affects the joints. Some studies have found a higher prevalence of SIBO in patients with rheumatoid arthritis, suggesting a possible relationship between both conditions.

Sjögren syndrome: Sjögren syndrome is an autoimmune disease that primarily affects the glands that produce tears and saliva. An increased incidence of SIBO has been observed in patients with Sjögren's syndrome.

Hashimoto thyroiditis: Hashimoto thyroiditis is an autoimmune disease that affects the thyroid gland. Some studies have suggested a possible association between SIBO and Hashimoto's thyroiditis.

The reasons behind the association between SIBO and autoimmune diseases are not fully elucidated, but several theories have been proposed. One of them is that bacterial overgrowth in the small intestine can affect the intestinal barrier and increase permeability, which could allow bacteria and their components to enter the bloodstream and trigger an autoimmune response. In addition, alteration of the intestinal microbiota in SIBO may influence immune regulation and trigger an unbalanced immune response.

The approach to SIBO in patients with autoimmune diseases may be more complex due to the presence of other conditions and the need to consider possible interactions between the drugs used to treat both conditions. A multidisciplinary approach and collaboration between gastroenterologists and immunologists may be necessary for optimal management in these cases.

Although the association between SIBO and autoimmune diseases is increasingly recognized, more research is needed to fully understand the nature of this relationship. The study of these interactions can provide valuable information to improve the clinical management and quality of life of patients with autoimmune diseases associated with SIBO.

SIBO AND NUTRIENT MALABSORPTION

The relationship between SIBO (Bacterial Overgrowth in Small Intestine) and nutrient malabsorption is an important and relevant connection in the field of gastrointestinal health. SIBO may adversely affect the ability of the small intestine to absorb nutrients adequately, which can lead to nutritional deficiencies and a range of health problems.

When bacterial overgrowth occurs in the small intestine, bacteria can compete with cells in the intestinal lining for nutrients, especially those that are easily fermented, such as nonabsorbable carbohydrates. In addition, bacteria in excess can damage intestinal epithelial cells and alter the structure of intestinal mucosa, decreasing the efficiency of nutrient absorption. This can lead to a number of malabsorption problems, including the following:

Fat malabsorption: Bacterial overgrowth can interfere with fat absorption in the small intestine. Bacteria can break down fats and produce secondary bile acids, reducing the availability of bile acids needed to emulsify fats and facilitate their absorption.

Carbohydrate malabsorption: Non-absorbable carbohydrates present in the diet, such as FODMAP (fermentable oligosaccharides, disaccharides, monosaccharides, and polyols), can be fermented by SIBO bacteria, resulting in the production of gases and liquids, and this can lead to gastrointestinal symptoms such as bloating, diarrhea, and abdominal distention.

Malabsorption of vitamins and minerals: SIBO can affect the absorption of certain vitamins and minerals, such as vitamin B12, vitamin D, iron, and calcium. Deficiency of these vitamins and minerals can have negative effects on general health and contribute to problems such as anemia and osteoporosis.

Protein malabsorption: Bacterial overgrowth can interfere with proper digestion and absorption of proteins, which can impair the supply of essential amino acids and contribute to muscle wasting and weakness.

Nutrient malabsorption associated with SIBO may cause gastrointestinal symptoms such as diarrhea, flatulence, bloating and fatty stools, as well as systemic symptoms such as fatigue, weakness, and specific nutritional deficiencies.

Management of SIBO and nutrient malabsorption usually involves addressing bacterial overgrowth by using specific antibiotics and/or dietary changes to reduce the burden of bacteria in the small intestine. In addition, nutritional supplements may be needed to correct vitamin and mineral deficiencies.

OTHER LINKS TO THE SIBO

In addition to the relationships mentioned above, SIBO (Small Intestine Bacterial Overgrowth) has been associated with other interesting links that deserve to be mentioned. These partnerships provide a more complete picture of the complexity and diversity of factors that can influence the development and course of the SIBO. Some of these other links are:

Intestinal dysbiosis refers to an imbalance in the composition of the intestinal microbiota, where certain bacterial species prevail over others. SIBO itself is a form of dysbiosis, involving abnormal overgrowth of bacteria in the small intestine. However, it has also been observed that generalized dysbiosis in the gastrointestinal tract may increase the risk of developing SIBO.

Alterations in intestinal motility, such as stagnation or slowing of intestinal transit, may predispose to the development of SIBO. Poor intestinal motility can allow bacteria to remain in the small intestine longer, making it easier for them to grow excessively.

Proton pump inhibitors (PPIs) and other drugs that reduce stomach acidity are commonly used to treat conditions such as heartburn and peptic ulcer disease. However, it has been observed that long-term use of these medicinal products may increase the risk of SIBO, as the acidic environment of the stomach is essential to control bacterial growth in the small intestine.

Obesity has been found to be associated with an increased risk of SIBO. The exact mechanisms are unclear, but alterations in intestinal motility, chronic inflammation, and the intestinal environment have been suggested to promote bacterial growth in people who are overweight or obese.

People who have had surgery to remove part of the small intestine, as in short bowel syndrome, may be at increased risk of SIBO because of reduced effective bowel length and changes in bowel motility.

Importantly, the relationship between SIBO and these links may vary by individual and the combination of factors present. In addition, some of these links can be both cause and consequence of the SIBO, making the relationship more complex and difficult to establish in all cases. Knowledge of these other links with SIBO is valuable for a better understanding of the pathophysiology of the disorder and for identifying potential risk factors.

TIPS FOR IMPROVING GUT HEALTH

LIFESTYLE HABITS FOR DIGESTIVE HEALTH

Lifestyle habits play a fundamental role in general digestive health, including prevention and management of SIBO (Small Intestine Bacterial Overgrowth). Adopting healthy habits can help maintain a balanced digestive system and promote an optimal gut environment for a healthy microbiota. Below are some lifestyle habits for digestive health:

Consuming a balanced diet rich in nutrients is essential for digestive health. Includes a variety of fruits, vegetables, lean protein, whole grains, and healthy fats. Dietary fiber is also important because it helps maintain adequate intestinal motility and promotes the health of the microbiota.

Proper chewing is the first step in the digestion process. By chewing food well, it facilitates the breakdown and assimilation of nutrients, reducing the burden on the digestive system.

Staying hydrated is essential for good bowel function. Water helps keep stools soft and promotes proper movement of the gastrointestinal tract.

Chronic stress can have a negative impact on the digestive system. Practicing stress management techniques, such as meditation, yoga, deep breathing, and regular physical activity, can help improve digestive health.

Regular exercise promotes bowel motility and helps prevent constipation and other digestive problems. In addition, exercise helps reduce stress and promote overall health.

Walking, an accessible, low-impact physical activity, offers multiple health benefits that accumulate over time, significantly improving overall physical well-being. This exercise, when incorporated regularly into the daily routine, can induce significant positive changes in several aspects of health.

First, walking improves cardiovascular health. As you walk, your heart works harder to pump blood to your moving muscles, which strengthens your heart muscle and improves blood circulation. This increase in heart activity helps to lower blood pressure and reduce the risk of cardiovascular diseases, such as heart attacks and strokes. Also, walking can help regulate blood cholesterol levels, increasing HDL (good) cholesterol and lowering LDL (bad) cholesterol, which is crucial to keeping arteries free of blockages.

Second, walking has a significant impact on body weight regulation and metabolism. This activity helps to burn calories, which is essential for weight control and obesity prevention. By walking regularly, the body improves its ability to handle insulin, which can prevent and help manage type 2 diabetes. Metabolism benefits from constant activity, maintaining a level of efficiency that facilitates the digestion and use of nutrients more effectively.

Also, walking benefits musculoskeletal health. Walking strengthens leg muscles, increases bone density, and improves joint flexibility and stability. This fortification of muscles and bones contributes to a lower risk of osteoporosis and arthritis and may decrease the likelihood of falls and fractures in older people. Walking also promotes better body posture and alignment, which can reduce aches and pains associated with poor posture or muscle conditions.

Walking not only directly influences physical health but also has positive effects on other aspects of well-being. For example, regular exercise, such as walking, has been associated with improvements in sleep quality and greater hormone balance, both of which are crucial for physical recovery and maintenance of health. In addition, being outdoors and walking, especially in natural environments, can increase exposure to sunlight, which is essential for the production of vitamin D, essential for bone health and immune function.

Heavy alcohol use and smoking can irritate the gastrointestinal mucosa and contribute to digestive problems. Reducing or avoiding these habits can be beneficial for digestive health.

Avoiding excessive alcohol consumption and smoking requires a multifaceted approach that includes awareness, self-discipline, and community support. Getting started with raising awareness of the health risks associated with these behaviors is a crucial step. Alcohol abuse and smoking are linked to a wide range of health problems, including cardiovascular disease, various cancers, liver, and respiratory problems, among others. Understanding these risks may motivate people to reduce or stop their use. In addition, setting clear and realistic personal goals for moderation or abstinence, and developing a detailed plan for achieving these goals, can provide the structure needed for change. This plan could include strategies such as limiting the amount of alcohol purchased or consumed, establishing alcohol and tobacco-free days, and avoiding situations or companies that encourage excessive drinking.

Social support plays a crucial role in the success of avoiding these harmful habits. Seeking support from friends, family, or support groups who understand and support the goal of living a life free of alcohol and tobacco can be tremendously beneficial. Engaging in activities and hobbies that do not revolve around the use of these substances can help reduce temptation and fill the time previously spent drinking or smoking. Also, in some cases, professional help, such as that of doctors, psychologists, or specialized support groups, may be needed to address underlying problems that contribute to alcohol abuse and smoking. Ultimately, a commitment to a healthy lifestyle, a willingness to seek and accept help when needed, and the development of positive coping strategies are critical to preventing excessive alcohol consumption and smoking.

Overuse of antibiotics may alter the gut microbiota and increase the risk of SIBO. Taking antibiotics only when needed and under the supervision of a health care practitioner is important.

Getting enough sleep and having a regular sleep schedule is important for digestive health. Proper sleep allows good repair and function of intestinal tissues.

Getting enough sleep and improving sleep quality are essential to overall health and well-being. Achieving a restful sleep begins with establishing a consistent routine, which involves lying down and waking up at the same time every day, including on weekends. This habit helps regulate the body's biological clock and facilitates a more predictable and satisfying sleep cycle. Creating an environment conducive to sleeping is equally important: the bedroom should be quiet, dark, and cool, and the bed comfortable. Minimizing exposure to electronic displays such as phones, tablets, and computers at least one hour before sleep can significantly improve sleep quality, because the blue light emitted by these devices can interfere with the production of melatonin, the hormone that regulates sleep.

Also, adopting relaxing bedtime practices can promote deeper, more restful sleep. Activities such as reading, deep breathing exercises, meditation, or gentle yoga can help calm the mind and prepare the body for rest. Attention to diet and exercise is also crucial: Avoiding caffeine and heavy meals in the hours before sleep can prevent interruptions of rest, while regular physical activity, preferably done in the morning or afternoon, can improve sleep quality and duration. By implementing these changes and maintaining a proactive attitude toward sleep hygiene, the foundations for more effective nights off can be laid, which in turn can improve physical and mental health, concentration, and overall quality of life.

Fast, processed foods are often low in nutrients and high in unhealthy fats and additives. These foods may be difficult to digest and may adversely affect digestive health.

Overweight and obesity can increase the risk of digestive problems, including SIBO. Maintaining a healthy weight through a balanced diet and regular exercise can promote digestive health.

By adopting these lifestyle habits, you can promote optimal digestive health and reduce the risk of gastrointestinal problems, including SIBO.

RECOMMENDED FOODS TO PROMOTE A HEALTHY MICROBIOTA

Promoting a healthy microbiota is essential to maintain good digestive health and prevent problems such as SIBO (Small Intestine Bacterial Overgrowth). A balanced and diverse gut microbiota plays a crucial role in digestion, nutrient absorption, immune function, and disease prevention. Here are some recommended foods to promote a healthy microbiota:

Foods rich in fiber: Food fibers are essential to feed beneficial bacteria in the gut. Fruits, vegetables, legumes, nuts, and seeds are excellent sources of fiber. Insoluble fibers promote proper movement of the gastrointestinal tract, while soluble fibers can help ferment and generate microbial beneficial short-chain fatty acids.

Fermented foods are rich in probiotics, which are beneficial bacteria that can colonize the gut and improve the balance of the microbiota. Examples include plain yogurt, kefir, sauerkraut, kimchi, tempeh, and miso.

Prebiotics: Prebiotics are specific types of fiber that act as food for beneficial bacteria in the intestine. Foods rich in prebiotics include artichokes, leeks, onions, garlic, asparagus, green bananas, and chicory, among others.

Healthy fats, such as those in olive oil, avocado, nuts, and seeds, can have a positive effect on the composition of the gut microbiota.

Antioxidants in fruits and vegetables, such as berries, spinach, and tomatoes, can help reduce inflammation and promote a bacteria-friendly gut environment.

Polyphenols are plant compounds with antioxidant and anti-inflammatory properties. They are found in foods such as green tea, cocoa, nuts, grapes, and blackberries and can contribute to a more diverse microbiota.

Foods rich in omega-3: Omega-3 fatty acids, present in fatty fish such as salmon, sardines, and nuts, may have a beneficial effect on gut health.

Choosing whole foods over highly processed versions can favor a healthier and more diverse microbiota.

Importantly, promoting a healthy microbiota is not only limited to the foods we eat, but also to our eating habits in general. Eating regularly and at consistent times, as well as chewing food well, are practices that can promote digestive health and microbiota.

It should be mentioned that each person is unique and can react differently to certain foods. Therefore, it is advisable to experiment and observe how the body feels with different foods to find the diet that best suits individual needs.

A balanced diet that includes high-fiber foods, prebiotics, probiotics, and antioxidants, along with a variety of healthy eating habits, can help promote a healthy microbiota and optimal digestive health.

STRATEGIES TO PREVENT RECURRENT SIBO

Preventing the recurrence of SIBO (Small Intestine Bacterial Overgrowth) is essential to maintain good digestive health and improve the quality of life of people who have experienced this condition. Recurrence of SIBO may occur, especially in people with underlying risk factors or who do not adequately address underlying triggers and causes. Here are some strategies that can help prevent SIBO recurrence:

Identifying and treating underlying causes: It is essential to identify and treat any underlying problems that may predispose to the development of SIBO. This can include intestinal motility disorders, autoimmune diseases, immune system dysfunction, among others. Working closely with a skilled health care practitioner can help address these causes and reduce the risk of recurrence.

Following appropriate treatment: If SIBO has been diagnosed and treated, it is important to follow the recommendations and treatment guidelines provided by a health care professional. This may include the use of specific antibiotics, changes in diet, and implementation of strategies to improve intestinal motility.

Adopt a personalized diet that avoids foods that can feed excessive bacterial growth and promote gut health. This may involve eliminating certain fermentable carbohydrates, known as FODMAP, for some people, while others may require a diet that is richer in fiber and prebiotics.

Supervise the use of acid inhibitors: If the use of proton pump inhibitors (PPIs) or other drugs that reduce stomach acidity is necessary, it should be done under the supervision of a health care professional and for the minimum necessary time. Reducing long-term use of these drugs can help maintain a more acidic gastric environment and prevent overgrowth of bacteria in the small intestine.

Supporting bowel motility: Strategies that promote adequate bowel motility can be useful in preventing SIBO recurrence. This may include the use of prokinetics, which are medicines that improve the movement of the gastrointestinal tract.

Probiotics: In some cases, selective use of probiotics may be beneficial in restoring and maintaining a healthy balance of the gut microbiota. However, it is important to use specific probiotics and under the supervision of a health care practitioner because certain probiotics can make SIBO worse in some people.

Stress management: Chronic stress can negatively affect gastrointestinal function and contribute to the development of SIBO. Stress management techniques, such as meditation, yoga, or cognitive-behavioral therapy, can help prevent SIBO recurrence.

Preventing recurrence of SIBO involves addressing the underlying causes, following appropriate treatment, and adopting a personalized approach that includes dietary changes, strategies to improve bowel motility, and stress management.

CONCLUSION

SIBO presents diagnostic and therapeutic challenges, highlighting the need to develop new management methods. Although progress has been made in understanding the gut microbiota, more research is needed to fully understand its pathophysiology. The standardization of diagnostic and therapeutic protocols is crucial for identifying biomarkers and specific treatments. Prioritizing professional medical consultation over self-diagnosis and self-medication is essential for the effective treatment of SIBO and related disorders.

In this journey through the world of digestive health and gut microbiota, we have learned that our digestive system is much more than just a process of assimilating food. It is a complex and dynamic ecosystem, where billions of bacteria work in harmony to keep us healthy and in balance.

Throughout these pages, we have explored in detail the SIBO and its impact on our digestive health. We have discovered its causes, risk factors, and how we can diagnose and treat it effectively. We have also understood their relationship with other health conditions and how our diet and lifestyle can influence their development and recurrence.

The key to maintaining a digestive system in balance and promoting a healthy microbiota lies in knowledge and action. We have learned that a balanced diet, rich in fiber and fermented foods, can nourish our beneficial bacteria and protect our gut health. In addition, we have found that minor changes in our lifestyle habits, such as managing stress and improving bowel motility, can have a significant impact on our digestive health.

It is important to remember that each of us is unique, and what works for one person may not be right for another. Therefore, it is essential to work together with health professionals to receive personalized care tailored to our individual needs.

This book has been a starting point for those seeking to understand and improve their digestive health. Our goal has been to demystify scientific concepts and provide practical tools to address SIBO and cultivate a healthy microbiota.

The path to optimal digestive health can be a challenge, but it is also a rewarding journey to a fuller and more vibrant life.

So, with the knowledge in hand and the power of action, I invite you to continue exploring and caring for your digestive health. May this book be just the beginning of a journey towards a healthier and more balanced life! Remember that digestive balance is the foundation for a full and radiant life!

RESOURCES

"The Gut Health Protocol: A Nutritional Approach To Healing SIBO, Intestinal Candida, GERD, Gastritis, and other Gut Health Issues" by John G. Herron

"SIBO: The Hidden Epidemic" por Dr. Allison Siebecker

Websites:

International Scientific Association for Probiotics and Prebiotics (ISAPP): https://isappscience.org/

National Institute of Diabetes and Digestive and Kidney Diseases (NIDDK): https://www.niddk.nih.gov/

The American Gastroenterological Association (AGA): https://gastro.org/

ABOUT SUSAN MCDOWELL

In the dynamic world of health and wellness, Dr. Susan McDowell stands out as a visionary and a beacon of knowledge, profoundly dedicated to empowering individuals to reach their full potential. Her journey in medicine is not merely a career, but a lifelong pursuit of understanding and sharing the intricacies of human well-being.

Dr. McDowell's foundational expertise was forged at the prestigious University of Medicine and Health Sciences, where she earned her medical degree. This rigorous academic background laid the groundwork for a professional path characterized by a unique blend of hands-on clinical expertise and an unwavering commitment to research. For years, she has cultivated her own medical practice, earning not only the respect but also the deep admiration of her patients through her compassionate care.

Beyond the clinic, Susan McDowell has forged an innovative path as a prolific writer, extending her influence far beyond individual consultations. Her extensive writings are a testament to her profound medical knowledge, yet they offer something more: they distill her innate compassion and unwavering dedication to continuously improving the health and well-being of all who seek her guidance. Her publications resonate deeply, reflecting an integrative approach that has made meaningful contributions to the field. While the sources don't specify all her topics, the mention of "Going barefoot" alongside her medical background hints at the breadth and diverse nature of her explorations within health and wellness, reflecting her prolific output.

Through both her clinical practice and her impactful written works, Susan McDowell has firmly established herself as a highly respected figure in the expansive field of health and medicine, a testament to her holistic vision and relentless dedication. She truly embodies the spirit of a leading medical professional, constantly pushing the boundaries of knowledge for the betterment of others.

Beyond her impressive credentials and extensive knowledge, Dr. Susan McDowell's approach to healthcare is deeply rooted in her profound empathy and a genuinely warm, welcoming demeanor. Her clinical practice is more than just a place for medical consultation; it is a space where her deep passion for helping people reach their full potential truly shines through. This innate drive translates into an environment where patients feel not just treated, but genuinely understood and cared for.

Dr. McDowell's personal philosophy distills her compassion and unwavering commitment to the continuous improvement of the health and well-being of those who seek her guidance. It is this patient-centered approach, marked by a welcoming spirit and an admirable dedication, that has earned her not just the respect, but the deep admiration of her patients over many years in her own practice. While the sources primarily highlight her interactions with patients and those who seek her guidance, her demonstrated compassion and dedication suggest an intrinsically warm and supportive professional persona.

OTHER BOOKS BY THE AUTHOR

"Andropause Exposed: The Hidden Male Menopause, Low Testosterone, and the Secret to Reclaiming Energy, Strength, and Confidence"

The groundbreaking book, "Andropause Exposed: The Hidden Male Menopause, Low Testosterone, and the Secret to Reclaiming Energy, Strength, and Confidence," offers a comprehensive, empathetic, and empowering guide to understanding, managing, and thriving through these changes.

"Parenting without fear: A Guide to Loving Your Children"

Are you tired of parenting approaches rooted in anxiety, control, or endless struggles? For generations, many parenting practices have been influenced by underlying fears: fear of children not learning, not behaving, or not succeeding. These methods, often relying on pressures, rewards, or anger, can be not only ineffective but also deeply detrimental to a child's intrinsic drive for self-development. In 'Parenting without Fear,' we invite you to embark on a revolutionary journey that challenges conventional wisdom and reconsiders the very foundation of how you guide your children.

"Going barefoot: natural running, walking and movement to respect your body"

In "Going Barefoot: Natural Running, Walking and Movement to Respect Your Body," Susan McDowell delves into the profound benefits of reconnecting with the earth through natural movement. This insightful book emphasizes the importance of barefoot activities in fostering alignment, strength, and overall well-being. Drawing from both scientific research and her rich clinical experience, Susan offers practical advice and exercises to help readers embrace a more natural way of moving.

"Understanding SIBO: The Enigma of Small Intestinal Bacterial Overgrowth".

This book, the result of Susan's clinical experience, offers a clear and practical perspective on Small Intestinal Bacterial Overgrowth Syndrome (SIBO). Through her work, Susan unravels the mysteries of this condition, providing readers with an essential guide to understanding, addressing, and overcoming SIBO.

"Understanding Perimenopause: A Woman in Plenitude"

Discover the beauty in every change, from hormonal aspects to symptoms and body changes. With personal stories and anecdotes that resonate, you will feel accompanied in this unique chapter of your life. It explores how sexual health, emotional and psychological aspects, and general well-being intertwine in a journey full of authenticity and self-acceptance.

"Complete Guide to Red Light Therapy: Optimal Health, Healthy Skin and Other Benefits of Red Light."

As an advocate of holistic approaches to health, Susan explores the diverse benefits of red-light therapy in this book. From improving skin health to optimizing overall wellness, Susan's comprehensive guide offers valuable information backed by research, allowing readers to effectively integrate red light into their daily routine.

"Microdosing: Macrobenefits in health and well-being. Your body in psychedelic and non-psychedelic substances."

In her most innovative work, Susan explores the fascinating world of microdosing and its impacts on health and wellness. This book provides a balanced and scientifically grounded view on the use of psychedelic and non-psychedelic substances in microdosing, offering a unique perspective on their potential benefit to mental and emotional health.

"High-Need Babies, The Untold Truth: The Ultimate Parenting Guide for High-Demanding Childs (English Edition)"

Susan McDowell embarks on the journey of parenting with her English-language play "High-Need Babies." This book provides a unique and comprehensive insight for parents facing the challenge of raising children with high demands. With empathy and wisdom, Susan guides parents through effective strategies and offers an enlightening perspective on the particular needs of these children.